Hormone Diet

Recharge Your Health, Balance Your Hormones, And Lose Weight with 18 Top Hormone Reset Diet Recipes

Introduction

Are you struggling to lose weight and/or lack energy or get tired every now and then while still struggling to stick to a 'diet'? If this best describes you, a hormone reset could be what you so desperately need.

Nowadays, when it comes to losing weight, you can only think of dieting because we've always been taught if you really want to shed off those extra pounds, you will need to restrict the amount of calories you consume per day.

But unfortunately, sheer willpower is simply not enough. The problem lies within your hormones.

The Hormone Reset Diet is a plan designed, specifically for women of all ages, sizes, shapes and races to lose weight and feel more energetic. There are certain foods that wreak havoc and develop resistance to your major metabolic hormones.

But by the end of three weeks, this guide will help you reverse hormone resistance, rebalance hormone receptors and enhance metabolism to kick start weight loss. By making simple dietary changes, you'll be able to shed pounds and feel livelier than you have in years.

Let's begin.

Thanks again for purchasing this book. I hope you enjoy it!

Table of Contents

Introduction _____ 2

How Do Hormones Make You Fat? _____ 7

    1: Estrogen _____ 8

    2: Insulin _____ 9

    3: Leptin _____ 9

    4: Testosterone _____ 11

    5: Thyroid Hormones _____ 11

    6: Cortisol _____ 12

    7: Melatonin _____ 13

    8: Ghrelin _____ 14

    9: Neuropeptide Y _____ 14

Step 1: Estrogen Reset _____ 16

    Self-assessment _____ 16

    How To Reset Estrogen _____ 18

Step 2: Insulin Reset _____ 20

    Self-Assessment _____ 20

    How To Reset Insulin Resistance _____ 22

Next, we will be focusing on resetting leptin levels. 28

Step 3: Leptin Reset 29
Self-Assessment 29
How To Reset Leptin Resistance 31

Step 4: Cortisol Reset 33
Self-Assessment 33
How To Reset Cortisol Immediately 34

Step 5: Thyroid Reset 35
Self-Assessment 35
How To Reset Thyroid 36

Step 6: Growth Hormone Reset 37
Self-Assessment 37
How To Reset Growth Hormone 38

Step 7: Testosterone Reset 39
Self-Assessment 39
How To Reset Testosterone 40

Hormone Reset Diet Recipes 42

Breakfast 42

Protein Egg Muffins _____ 42

Pumpkin Porridge _____ 44

Collagen Frappe And Tea _____ 45

Tulsi Tea _____ 46

Carrot Cake Muffins _____ 47

Cabbage Hash Browns _____ 49

Keto Cereal _____ 50

Main Meals _____ 52

Pistachio Crusted Stuffed Chicken Breasts _____ 52

Kale Pesto With Squoodles (Spaghetti Squash) _____ 55

Avocado, Quinoa And Garbanzo Bean Salad _____ 57

Avocado Chickpea Tuna Salad _____ 58

Ground Turkey Endive Roll-Ups _____ 60

Pistachio Crusted Peruvian Sea Bass And Maca ___ 62

Ceviche _____ 64

Crispy Sweet Potato Wedges _____ 66

Honey Garlic Glazed Salmon _____ 68

Hormone Reset Crab Cakes _____ 70

Cauliflower Fried Rice _____ 72

Chicken Parm Stuffed Peppers _____ 74

Desserts — 76

- Almond Butter Fudge Bars — 76
- Chia Seed Dessert — 78
- Hormone Reset Brownies — 79

Hormone Reset Dips — 81

- Creamy Dairy Free Brie — 81
- Spicy Mung-Bean Hummus — 83
- Cashew Cream Cheese — 84

Conclusion — 85

References — 86

Before we get to discuss how to reset your hormones for weight loss, let's first start by learning how hormones result to weight loss in the first place.

How Do Hormones Make You Fat?

Let me start by defining hormones.

Hormones are simply molecules or 'special chemical messengers' (that are secreted by special glands e.g. the thyroid glands) within the body's endocrine system.

Their function is to regulate various biological activities such as water and electrolyte balance, energy use and storage, reproduction, development and growth.

Many of these hormones are transported by the circulatory system to different parts of the body where they influence the cells as required.

However, specific hormones only influence the target cells that have receptors for each specific hormone. Therefore, when a hormone binds to a **receptor**, some change occurs within the cell to cause a particular cellular function to take place. This entire process is termed as **hormone signaling.** This process is very efficient and effective when it is working well i.e. when you are said to be experiencing hormonal balance.

Sometimes however, hormonal balance is disrupted by poor lifestyle choices and this ultimately leads to unhealthy weight gain. Below are the major metabolic hormones and how their imbalance results in weight gain.

1: Estrogen

This is one of two primary sex hormones for the female gender and is produced in the ovarian cells. Any imbalance, whether high or low, in the levels of estrogen will cause weight gain.

High levels of estrogen can result when you consume a diet that is rich in estrogen e.g. red meat. Nowadays, beef cattle are fed with synthetic estrogen compounds that enhance their feeding efficiency and enable them to pack on more weight. Consuming such meat from the animal increases estrogen levels in your body and this stresses the cells that produce insulin in your body.

You therefore end up becoming insulin resistant and blood sugar levels go high and then you end up gaining weight.

Women who are at their premenopausal stage are at great risk. This is the stage where the ovarian cells produce less estrogen. Since there isn't enough supply of estrogen anymore, the body resorts to other sources such as fat cells. When estrogen is low, the body begins to convert all the available sources of energy to fat so as to replenish glucose levels. Eventually, you end up gaining weight especially in the lower abdomen area.

Women between the ages of 35 and 50 are the ones at the highest risk since their ovaries secrete less progesterone and thus allowing estrogen to dominate.

2: Insulin

This hormone is secreted by the pancreas and its function is to help carry glucose into the cells so that it can be used as energy or to be converted and stored as fat. In short, insulin helps maintain a healthy level of glucose in the blood.

Blood sugar increases as you eat. To avoid the glucose levels going beyond normal, insulin lowers it from the bloodstream by directing it into 3 different organs of your body. First of all, a little amount of the glucose is directed to the liver, most of it is used up by the muscles as fuel and the surplus is converted and stored as fat.

But in some instances, due to poor lifestyle choices and diet, such as binging on processed foods and drinks, taking artificially sweetened drinks and snacking leads to insulin resistance.

This is a phenomenon where the cell receptors no longer sense the presence of insulin, even though it is there in overabundance. This means that muscle cells are no longer aware of the glucose bound insulin thus, glucose levels keep increasing in the bloodstream. This spike in blood sugar levels leads to Type 2 diabetes and a sudden weight gain.

3: Leptin

Leptin (usually referred to as the satiety hormone) is a hormone that is secreted from stored fat cells of the white adipose tissues. This means that the amount of leptin in your bloodstream is directly proportionate to the total amount of body fat. Therefore, the more fat you have, the greater the amount of leptin you produce.

Leptin is the most important hormone when it comes to understanding your sensation of hunger and satiety. When it is produced in high quantities, it signals the brain to tell you that you are full and you should stop eating. When its level drops, you start feeling hungry and you begin to crave for food.

People who are overweight or obese have more body fat in their fat cells than required. Since it is the fat cells that secrete leptin in proportion to the amount of body fat, such persons produce very high amounts of leptin. Considering the way in which leptin functions, and given the brain knows that the body has more than enough energy reserves, such people shouldn't actually eat.

The problem therefore is that the brain no longer senses the presence of leptin, even though it is there in excess. This phenomenon is what is called **leptin resistance.**

Leptin resistance therefore occurs when your body is continuously overexposed to high levels of leptin and it eventually affects your brain's sensitivity to leptin. When your body becomes resistant to leptin, it may require a much higher quantity of leptin before the brain signals the body that you feel full. So obese persons have abnormally high leptin levels but they are unresponsive to it.

4: Testosterone

This steroidal hormone is produced by both humans and animals. It is a predominantly male sex hormone although females secrete it too in small amounts. This is the hormone responsible for increased bone density, muscle mass, libido, facial hair and even deep voice. In short, testosterone is necessary for a healthy body and plays a critical role in metabolism.

Studies show that people with low testosterone have a higher percentage of body fat as compared to people with higher quantities of testosterone. This means that a dip in testosterone levels causes an increase in body weight especially in the midsection (and the opposite is true).

Stress and age are some of the reasons behind low production of testosterone. Inadequate exercise, irregular sleep patterns and poor diet are other causes. Being overweight hampers your ability to produce enough testosterone and lowers the already low testosterone level in the body and this can become a vicious cycle.

5: Thyroid Hormones

These hormones are produced by a butterfly shaped gland known as the thyroid gland that is located at the back of your neck. The 3 most active thyroid hormones produced are thyroxine (T4), triiodothyronine (T3) and calcitonin. These three work together to regulate your body's metabolic functioning, bone maintenance, mood regulation, brain development, muscle control as well as heart and digestive functions.

Underproduction (hypothyroidism) of these thyroid hormones is strongly associated with gaining weight. As a matter of fact, sudden weight gain is one of the most common signs that the thyroid is not producing enough hormones.

A poor diet or malnutrition, physical inactivity and stress are some of the reasons for an underperforming thyroid. Others include environmental toxins and gluten intolerance. It is also said that hypothyroidism also leads to accumulation of water in the body, making a patient appear plump.

6: Cortisol

Cortisol (popularly known as the stress hormone) is a steroid hormone that is secreted by the adrenal glands, which are endocrine glands found just above the kidney. It is a fight or flight hormone that is secreted when you are stressed out, anxious, depressed, angry, nervous or physically injured. It is produced so as to replenish energy you expend after fleeing from or fighting a perceived threat.

Poor lifestyle choice such as inadequate sleep also makes your body be in a constant state of stress.

But too often, the modern human being usually responds to stress by stewing and sitting in anger, sadness or frustration without using up any energy that you would have if you were physically fleeing or fighting your way from a wild beast hunting you down (like our ancestors so often did).

Therefore, when you are seated there lost in stressful thoughts, your neuroendocrine system thinks that you are physically fleeing or fighting. Cortisol is still released into your system whether or not your stressor requires you to respond physically or emotionally.

For some individuals, cortisol runs through their bodies almost constantly since their typical day has no break from stress. This makes their bodies' hyperinsulinemic and increases the deposition of fat on the body. This constantly elevated cortisol also leaves you vulnerable to developing diabetes, high blood pressure and lowers your immunity in general.

7: Melatonin

To maintain the body's internal clock (sleeping and rising time), melatonin is secreted by the pineal gland, a pea-shaped gland located in the brain. Secretion of melatonin happens more during the night because light has been found to somehow hinder the production of this hormone. This means that melatonin levels are lowest during daytime.

Researchers have found that there is a link between low levels of melatonin and a tendency to put on weight. Getting some quality bedtime is not easy when not enough melatonin is being produced.

Whenever you keep disrupting the circadian rhythm either because there isn't enough darkness around or for some reason you cannot get enough sleep, you increase the production of ghrelin, leptin and cortisol. Once these hormones are elevated, you end up gaining weight and you also make losing the weight way more difficult.

The production of melatonin is very low between the ages of 6 and 20 but then steadies between 20s and 40s after which, it begins to drop again once you've gone past the 40 age mark.

8: Ghrelin

Also known as the hunger hormone, ghrelin is produced mainly by the stomach and its work is to stimulate appetite and also plays a role in deposition of fat. When your stomach is empty, ghrelin is secreted to send a signal to the hypothalamus and trigger hunger, telling you that it's time to eat. The pancreas, brain and small intestines also produce ghrelin but in smaller quantities.

Thus, ghrelin levels are high just before you eat and lowest when you have eaten. However, in overweight people, ghrelin levels are abnormally lower than in people of normal weight.

After an overweight person has finished eating, ghrelin only drop off slightly. The hypothalamus therefore fails to receive as strong message as it should to stop you from eating and you end up overfeeding.

9: Neuropeptide Y

NPY is secreted by cells in the nervous system and the brain. It is an appetite stimulant and once in the system, you specifically crave for carbohydrates.

Neuropeptide is at its peak when you are deprived of food or when you are fasting. It will usually stick a bit longer when you are going through periods of stress, which can cause binge eating and eventually fat gain.

Now that you have a good understanding of how different hormones affect weight loss, the next thing you might be wondering is how to reset different hormones to ultimately reverse weight gain. That's what we will be discussing next.

Step 1: Estrogen Reset

The first step to losing weight is resetting your out of balance estrogen, a state where you have too much estrogen compared to the counter-hormone progesterone. To start off, you will need to assess yourself to determine whether estrogen is one of the reasons you are struggling with weight loss.

Self-assessment

In the last few months, have you been experiencing some of the following problems?

- Gallbladder problems

- Rapid weight gain that is proving difficult to lose especially in the butt and hip region.

- Frequent blushing or a red flush on your face caused when you use dairy, spicy foods, red wine, skin products or when there's a lot of heat?

- Anxiety, mini breakdowns (over the most ridiculous things), irritability, mood swings, depression etc.

- Painful periods, endometriosis, fibroids, postmenopausal bleeding or heavy bleeding

- Breast tenderness and/or increased size of bra-cup

- Autoimmune conditions (when your own immune system launches an attack on your body tissues) e.g. Thyroiditis (Hashimoto's disease)

- Soreness in the LV3 point (hollow located between your second toe and the big toe somewhere on top of your foot especially when you massage the area) which is a symptom of estrogen dominance.
- Fluid retention or bloating

You are likely to be estrogen dominant if you have five or more of the signs listed above. If so, no need to panic, as we will be addressing this hormone imbalance situation immediately by following the instructions.

How To Reset Estrogen

To reset estrogen, there are two key tips you need to keep in mind. You have to abstain from anything with alcohol or meat in it while also increasing fiber intake, which will boost weight loss. It's really quite that easy.

Consume at least one pound of vegetables per day divided over 2 or 3 three meals depending on your meal frequency. A pound of vegetables is equivalent to 5 to 10 cups. Of course, this will depend on the type of vegetables or whether they're cooked or raw. Don't forget to eat the healthy proteins (eggs, chicken, shellfish, sardines, mackerel, tilapia, salmon and cod).

Also, your fiber consumption should increase by 5 grams per day to a favorable range of 35 to 45 grams each day. More fiber improves the ability of your liver to take out excess estrogen. This means that when you increase fiber intake, you expel more estrogen from the body. Don't be tempted by the overabundance of packaged foods written 'rich in fiber' in the stores. Just stick to the fiber that you acquire from plants. Most of these packaged foods with added fiber such as bread have plenty of salt, sugar and other chemicals you don't want to be consuming. The best fiber rich foods are legumes, lentils, organic vegetables, flax seeds and chia seeds. You can also take fiber powders and capsules.

Since you've given up meat, you are presented with the opportunity to fill up on healthy fats. Eat unprocessed natural fats found in whole foods. For cooking, use healthy saturated fats such as virgin red palm oil and coconut oil since both add flavor to food and are also stable at high temperatures.

Eat monounsaturated fats found in nut and nut butter, duck fat, dark chocolate and avocados. Polyunsaturated fats can be found in pastured poultry and eggs, sunflower, chia and flax seeds, all nuts and nut oils (almonds, walnuts, pine nuts etc), clarified butter, pastured ghee evening primrose and borage oil, crustaceans (crab, shrimp and oysters) and fish (mackerel, halibut and salmon).

Step 2: Insulin Reset

The most common hormonal reason for weight gain and weight metabolism is developing resistance to insulin.

Self-Assessment

To determine whether you are insulin resistant, check which of the following signs and symptoms have occurred to you in the recent past or apply to you.

- If you have a fasting insulin level that is more than 5 micro units per milliliter

- If your blood pressure is high i.e. 140 or above for the systolic and 90 and above for the diastolic

- If you have low triglycerides i.e. low good HDL cholesterol

- You feel cranky or fatigued when you skip a meal or when you go hungry

- If you gain weight aggressively or with a lot of ease and cannot find a solution on how to lose it.

- If you suffer form (PCOS) polycystic ovary syndrome. This is a condition that is characterized by cysts on the ovaries, increased growth of hair, acne, irregular periods and sometimes infertility

- If your body mass index is more than 25. To determine your BMI, divide your weight in kilograms against height in square meters (m²).

- If your waist from the belly button measures 35 inches or more for ladies and 40 for men.

- If you feel irritable, anxious and shaky after going for three hours or more without eating or if you crave for junk food to calm you down.

- If your blood sugar level is higher than it should i.e. if it is higher than 85 milligrams per deciliter.

- If you have tried before to quit eating candies and other sweet stuff without any degree of success i.e. you can't stop eating foods packed in carbs such as ice cream, chocolate or even French fries.

You are very likely to be insulin resistant if you have 5 or more of the above symptoms and at significant risk of developing pre-diabetes and diabetes.

How To Reset Insulin Resistance

Eliminate Sugar

It is very possible to reset your insulin pathway within 3 days if you strictly adhere to this guide. The very first thing to do here is to eliminate sugar and sugar related substitutes from your diet.

You know all the usual suspects here: soda, muffins, doughnuts, cookies. Cutting back on sugar also includes the sugar substitutes as well (apart from Stevia).

Avoid the following sugary substances: molasses, maple syrup, splenda (sucralose), brown sugar, agave, honey, and white table sugar. There are other substances that contain hidden sugars. You will need to avoid these; packaged cereals, sauces, salad dressings and ketchup.

The American Heart Association recommends 25 grams of sugar per day but in this case, you will only be taking 15 grams per day, 10 grams less. Therefore, the next time you scrutinize product labels when you go out for shopping, look out for the grams of sugar. This will enable you to choose products that contain little amounts of sugar.

Watch the amount of food you eat

It is also important to watch the amount of food you eat. While the pancreas secretes differing amounts of insulin depending on the type of food you consume, eating a large portion size in one sitting can cause hyperinsulinemia (having high levels of insulin in the body). This is true especially if you are an overweight person with insulin resistance.

In a study, it was observed that obese people struggling with insulin resistance who were made to eat a 1,300 calorie meal had double the amount of insulin as people with normal weight who had the same meal. On the contrary, having fewer calories has consistently shown to reduce insulin levels and improve insulin sensitivity among overweight people regardless of the food they eat.

Reduce the amount of carbs from your diet

Out of all three macronutrients (fat, carbs and protein), carbohydrates are the ones that raise insulin and blood sugar levels the most. This is the reason why you will want to cut back on carb rich foods.

Did you know that a low carb diet is very effective if you want to lose weight? Studies show that a carb restricted diet has the ability to enhance insulin sensitivity and reduce insulin levels way more than other diets. In one study for instance, persons suffering from metabolic syndrome were divided into two groups. One group was given a low carb diet and the other was given a low fat diet. Both diets amounted up to 1500 calories each.

It was discovered that insulin levels had dropped by an average of 50% for the low carb patients as compared to only 19% for the low fat patients.

Include apple cider vinegar in your diet

Apple cider vinegar prevents sharp rises in insulin and blood sugar after you have eaten. This is true especially when the apple cider vinegar comes after you've had a meal containing high carbohydrates. Scientists believe that this usually happens since vinegar has the ability to delay stomach emptying. And thus this leads to a slower absorption of glucose into the bloodstream. A study found that persons who ingested 28 ml (about 2 tablespoons) of vinegar after eating a high carb diet exhibited greater feelings of satiety and lower insulin levels.

Green tea

Tests show that green tea contains high amounts of an antioxidant known as epigallocatechin gallate (EGCC), which apparently reverses insulin resistance.

In one study for example, patients suffering from abnormally high insulin levels were made to drink green tea for half a year. They reported to have a decrease in insulin after that period.

Soluble fiber

This type of fiber dissolves in the presence of water to form a gel-like substance that slows down food movement through the digestive tract. This leaves you feeling satiated. It also keeps the blood sugar and insulin in check after you've eaten.

Moreover, friendly bacteria living in your colon feed off soluble fiber. In turn, they decrease insulin resistance and improve your overall gut health.

Women who eat the biggest amount of soluble fiber have a 50% chance of becoming insulin resistant, as compared to women who had the smallest amount of soluble fiber. This is according to an observational study.

Avoid physical inactivity

There's no way you can reverse insulin sensitivity when you lead a sedentary lifestyle either at home or at work. A study conducted among middle aged sedentary ladies that took half a year showed that the ladies that went for a walk for 20 minutes after a huge meal were reported to have improved insulin sensitivity as compared to women who never took in the walk after eating.

The group that walked also lost a considerable amount of body fat and became fitter. It was therefore right to conclude that walking around or doing some sort of physical activity rather than just sitting for a long time can keep insulin levels from spiking once you have eaten.

The best exercises to decrease insulin are resistance training for sedentary and older adults and aerobic exercises for people with type-2 diabetes and the obese.

Eliminate refined carbs from your diet

In this age, refined carbs make a huge chunk of our diet. But this shouldn't be the case since consuming them regularly presents a number of health hazards. Among those problems are obesity and high insulin levels.

Such refined carbs are said to have a high glycemic index (GI). This is a scale that measures the ability of a certain type of food to raise blood sugar. The glycemic load takes into consideration the amount of digestible carbs found in a single serving as well as the glycemic index.

Studies have been conducted to compare different foods containing different glycemic loads to determine whether they varying effects on insulin levels. Consuming a food that is high on glycemic load was found to spike insulin levels way more than consuming the same amount of food but with a low glycemic load even when the carb contents of the two foods are the same.

It is therefore important to replace refined carbs which are digested and absorbed quicker with carbs that are digested a lot slower, as this may help bring down insulin levels.

Such foods are: semolina, freekeh, buckwheat, couscous, pearl, barley, quinoa, brown rice, long grain, doongora and basmati rice, rice noodles, soba noodles, pasta, yams, corn, sweet potatoes, Nicola and Carisma potato varieties, zucchini, cauliflower, celery, broccoli, carrots, bircher muesli, oats, bran, sourdough bread, rye and whole grain bread., almond milk, soy milk, custard, beans, peas, lentils and kiwi.

Use cinnamon

Cinnamon is a sweet smelling and delicious spice that is packed with health boosting antioxidants. Studies show that patients with insulin resistance and healthy people who use this spice can decrease insulin levels and improve insulin sensitivity.

In a small study, young people who drank liquids containing a lot of sugar were still able to experience lower insulin levels after using cinnamon for the entire 14 days than when they drank the high sugar liquids and taking a placebo.

In a different study, healthy persons who ate rice pudding with 1 ½ teaspoons of cinnamon in it had considerably lower insulin responses than people who had eaten rice pudding without cinnamon.

Eat the right amount and type of protein

Including sufficient protein in your diet can help you control insulin levels and your weight as well. However, protein can sometimes increase the secretion of insulin so that your muscles can absorb amino acids. This is the reason why you should avoid consuming high amounts of proteins since they lead to increased insulin production.

Moreover, there are some proteins that stimulate greater insulin response than others. For instance, casein and whey protein both found in dairy products have been found to raise insulin levels a lot more even than bread does when consumed by healthy people.

The best protein you can consume if you want to solve insulin issues are those from fatty fish such as anchovies, herring, mackerel, sardines and salmon. Apart from providing you with high quality protein, they are also the best sources of long chain omega-3 fatty acids you will find around.

And studies show that fatty fish can help bring down insulin resistance especially if you are suffering from PCOS (polycystic ovary syndrome), gestational diabetes or obesity. In one study, a woman suffering from PCOS recorded a remarkable 8.4% decrease in insulin levels after she took fish oil. In another study, some adolescents and obese children took fish supplements and thereafter, they were found to have significantly low levels of triglycerides (bad cholesterol) and insulin resistance.

Next, we will be focusing on resetting leptin levels.

Step 3: Leptin Reset

Self-Assessment

Use the following to determine whether you have developed resistance to leptin:

- ✓ High triglycerides of more than 100 mg/Dl

- ✓ Joint problems such as joint pains, arthritis, bursitis. Or perhaps your doctor suggested that you undergo shoulder, hip or knee surgery.

- ✓ Fatigue after working out or difficulty completely recovering

- ✓ Profuse and weird sweating patterns compared with how it was a couple of years ago

- ✓ Increased fat deposits around the triceps muscles on your arm (kimono arms)

- ✓ Menopausal weight gain more so at the waistline

- ✓ Obesity or excess weight (body mass index exceeding 25) especially if you are more than 30 pounds your normal weight.

- ✓ If you love drinking more than one serving of sodas or fruit juices per day.

- ✓ If you have a tendency to wait an hour or longer or skipping breakfast entirely after waking up

- ✓ A strong and occasionally voracious desire for food

- ✓ Cold body temperatures which are less than 36°C or 98°F.
- ✓ Reduced sex drive and infertility
- ✓ Slow resting heart rate (below 60) which is a result of poor aerobic conditioning and being overweight or obese.
- ✓ If the optimum serum leptin level is more than 10 – 12.

You are likely to be leptin resistant if you have 5 or more of the above symptoms.

How To Reset Leptin Resistance

Eliminate fructose from your diet

Fructose is a natural simple sugar found in honey, fruits and vegetables as well as food and drink sweeteners such as high fructose corn syrup (HCFS). Fructose is also the major component in brown sugar, table sugar, agave, maple syrup and molasses. Omitting fructose can improve leptin and insulin resistance, the best case scenario of killing two birds with one stone.

A recent research study conducted by scientists from the University of Florida and published in the American Journal of Physiology – Regulatory, Integrative and Comparative Physiology showed how diets high in fructose caused leptin resistance in rats and that eventually made them become overweight.

The rats were divided into two groups. For a period of 6 months, the first group was fed with diets that did not contain any fructose while the other group was fed with a diet that comprised of 60% fructose.

When the period was over, the rats were tested for leptin. It was found that the rats that were fed with a 60% fructose diet had developed resistance to leptin. Surprisingly, the same rats also had higher levels of **triglycerides** in their bloodstream than their counterparts. In the other group of rats, there was no significant change in the levels of leptin, insulin, glucose and cholesterol.

Afterwards, the scientists isolated half the number of rats from each group and they were fed a high fat diet for a fortnight. The rats that were earlier on a 60% fructose diet were seen to increase their amount of food consumption and consequently put on more weight than rats that were on a fructose free diet. This made the scientists to conclude that the epidemic of obesity is worsened by diets that combine high amounts of fructose with high amounts of fats and calories.

From this study, there are two ways in which fructose has been shown to affect the leptin pathways. The first is that high fructose on its own promptly renders the hypothalamus resistant to leptin. Normal functioning receptors in the hypothalamus seem to become muted and ineffective in the presence of leptin when fructose level in the blood is high. Secondly, consumption of fructose results in the body producing a lot of triglycerides. Triglycerides have been shown to block the passage of leptin to the brain. This study shows that triglycerides promote leptin resistance by impairing leptin transport across the BBB (blood brain barrier) and so not enough leptin gets to the receptors in the brain to produce the desired effect.

Step 4: Cortisol Reset

Self-Assessment

You have to reset your cortisol if the following conditions or behaviours apply to you:

- If you have premenstrual syndrome
- If you have fibrocystic breast change or if you experience breast tenderness
- If you have osteoporosis, osteopenia or have thinning bones
- If you regularly suffer from stomach ulcers, gastroesophagial reflux disease or indigestion
- If you suffer from burnout i.e. emotional or physical exhaustion due to chronic stress
- If you are addicted to coffee
- If you overeat when stressed
- If you drink more than three servings of alcohol every week
- If you struggle with irritability or anxiety
- If you have difficulty sleeping at night

How To Reset Cortisol Immediately

Eliminate caffeine

Do away with all coffee and caffeinated products such as energy drinks, soda, green tea and black tea for good. Replace these with much healthier alternatives such as mushroom teas, herbal teas, hot water with cardamom, hot water with cayenne and lemon etc.

Exercise regularly

Studies conducted by scientists from Harvard Medical School show that half an hour to a full hour of exercise a few times per week is the best way to manage stress by balancing cortisol levels. This enables you to normalize metabolic functions and sleep better. However, it is important not to overdo the exercises as they can cause even more cortisol to be secreted.

Step 5: Thyroid Reset

Self-Assessment

The next step is for you to complete a self assessment to determine the extent of your thyroid issues. Have you experienced or do you have the following:

- Autoimmune condition or Hashimoto's disease?
- Restless legs syndrome?
- Difficulty walking due to either loss of coordination or balance? Or even walking with a wide gait?
- Unexplained and repeated miscarriages, menstrual disorders or infertility?
- Mineral and/or vitamin deficiencies?
- Skin rashes, acne, eczema and hair loss?
- Chronic fatigue or brain fog?
- Bone pain, joint aches?
- Autism, attention deficit??
- Weight gain, stubborn fat (difficulty in losing weight)
- Headaches and migraines?
- Schizophrenia, depression and anxiety?

- Diarrhea and constipation, food poisoning, smelly gas, abdominal bloating and pain?

If you have 5 or more of these symptoms, there is a big chance that you are suffering from a thyroid hormone problem, which needs to be reset.

How To Reset Thyroid

Eliminate all foods made from grain, including flour. Avoid foods such as rice, millet, spelt, durum, corn, oats, barley, rye and wheat and any other byproducts made from any of these grains.

Do away with processed foods that contain grain, thickeners or gluten derivatives. Such include are spices, beer, cream sauces, pasta, bread, pizza, processed cheeses, nondairy creamers, dried soup mixes, canned soups, salad dressings, ice cream, pickles, mustard, luncheon meats and hot dogs.

As a substitute for grains, you can eat kelp noodles, baked sweet potatoes, coconut flour, romaine lettuce, dehydrated vegetable crackers, flaxseed crackers, yams, roasted seaweed and coconut wraps.

Step 6: Growth Hormone Reset

Naturally, milk contains growth hormones and this explains why it is the only food for young ones. However, most dairy cows are injected with genetically modified growth hormones so that they may produce more milk than how they would when normal. And when you consume this milk, you too introduce these hormones into your body which can wreck your hormonal ecosystem.

Self-Assessment

If you may have experienced the following within the past few months, you might need to reset your growth hormones:

- Anaphylaxis, a severe and allergic reaction that causes swelling, which can make it difficult for you to either swallow, talk or breathe.
- Sinus infection
- Addiction to cheese or milk-based treats such as frappuccino or latte
- Skin reactions such as red skin, hives, itchy bumps, rash etc.
- Wheezing, sneezing, coughing, gurgling belly, itchy and watery eyes, runny or stuffy nose especially after eating yogurt
- Irritable bowel or bloating
- Swelling of the mouth, throat, face, tongue or lips.

How To Reset Growth Hormone

Avoid all dairy related products including milk itself, yogurt, kefir, butter and cheese. However, there are some great alternatives to dairy including coconut kefir, hemp milk, coconut milk, and almond milk. After you have done away with dairy, you will have plenty of room to consume alkaline forming foods such as vegetables that are rich in iron, minerals and fiber.

Step 7: Testosterone Reset

Self-Assessment

Have you or do you experience the following:

- Bad breath?
- Heartburn, burping, nausea, bloating and gas in the tummy
- Irritability, anxiety, depression and mood swings
- Water retention that causes a puffy looking face
- Poor memory or brain fog
- Mucus in the eyes or itchy eyes when you wake up
- Eye bags or dark circles around the eyes
- Dry skin, rashes or hives, tinnitus or itching ears
- Chest congestion or bronchitis and colds
- Achy joints
- Fatigue even after sleeping for 8 hours straight

If you've experienced several of these symptoms, you most likely have a problem with testosterone that needs to be corrected. Here is how to go about it.

How To Reset Testosterone

Use safe food containers

Avoid storing food or warming food in plastic. Use stainless steel or glass.

Increase intake of alkaline-forming foods

The best way to achieve this is to begin your day by having a cup of hot water with lemon and then a green shake or smoothie for breakfast. Ensure that you consume around 2 or 3 servings or greens daily. Also eat 35 to 45 grams of fiber per day to help bind metabolic blockers.

Look out for toxic products

Ensure anything that you use or apply is free from metabolic blockers. Use only biodynamic lotions and soaps, natural conditioners and shampoos and organic deodorant and toothpaste.

Get out more often

Did you know that according to the Environmental Protection Agency, the air you breathe inside your house could be more than 5 times more polluted than what you'll find outside? This is why you'll need to go outdoors more often, put casings on mattresses and pillows and run a HEPA filter.

Now that you've learned how to reset different hormones, I know you might be wondering how to go about resetting different hormones with your diet. The truth is, you may be having several hormonal problems at the same time, which means you cannot just reset one hormone at a time while wreaking havoc on another. That's why the next part of the book will focus on recipes you can prepare to help you to reset all your hormones holistically through taking the right dietary choices.

Hormone Reset Diet Recipes

Breakfast

Protein Egg Muffins

Serves 12

Ingredients

½ pound shredded or chopped (into small pieces) and fully cooked chicken breast, bacon or sausage

¼ cup of finely shallots or green onions

1 teaspoon of cayenne pepper

½ teaspoon of fennel seeds

½ teaspoon of black pepper

½ teaspoon of salt

12 large eggs

1 cup of shredded chard

1 minced garlic clove

1 teaspoon of coconut oil

Directions

1. Preheat the oven to 218.3°C (425°F).

2. Heat the coconut oil in a large frying pan over medium heat. Toss in the garlic and cook for a few minutes until it gets soft.

3. Toss in the chard then cover the frying pan with a tight fitting lid. Let this cook for 3 minutes or so until the chard becomes tender and appears brighter. Strain it then rinse it with cold water and set aside.

4. Beat all eggs in large bowl and add the cayenne, fennel seeds, pepper and salt then stir in the onions and chard.

5. Line 12 paper baking cups on a muffin tin. Fill each cup halfway with the mixture above. Scoop a few tablespoons of the chopped chicken breast, bacon or sausage onto each cup. Add some more of the egg mixture to seal the muffin.

6. Put the muffins in the oven and bake for about 35 minutes or until the egg turns golden brown on the muffin top.

Pumpkin Porridge

Serves 1

Ingredients

Xylitol or Stevia

1 to 4 tablespoons of unsweetened coconut milk

2 tablespoons of shredded coconut

½ teaspoon of cinnamon

½ cup of pumpkin puree

1 tablespoon of tahini

1 tablespoon of finely ground Marcona almonds

3 tablespoons of finely ground hemp seeds

1 tablespoon of casein free pastured ghee

Directions

1. Put the ghee in a small pan and heat it over low heat.
2. Toss in the rest of the ingredients while adjusting the coconut milk so that you achieve your preferred consistency and keep stirring.
3. Serve porridge while warm.

Collagen Frappe And Tea

Serves 1

Ingredients

1 tablespoon of MCT oil

3 tablespoons of clean protein (collagen)

Brewed tea

Directions

Put all 3 ingredients in a blender and blend for half a minute or so then serve

Tulsi Tea

Serves 2 or 3

Ingredients

4 cups of cool water

4 cups of boiling water

4 tablespoons of dried dandelion leaves

8 tablespoons of dried organic tulsi

Directions

1. Immerse the dandelion and Tulsi leaves in the boiling water and let it soak for at least half an hour.

2. Once the tea is saturated to your liking, strain the leaves and add cool water.

3. Serve the tea. It is usually served at room temperature

Carrot Cake Muffins

Serves 18

Ingredients

½ cup of chopped walnuts

¼ cup of oats

2 cups of shredded carrots

¼ cup of plain Greek yogurt

½ cup of unsweetened apple sauce

2 teaspoons of vanilla extract

3 large eggs

1 cup of light brown sugar

¾ cup of melted coconut oil

¼ teaspoon of ground ginger

¼ teaspoon of nutmeg

1 teaspoon of cinnamon

½ teaspoon of salt

2 teaspoons of baking soda

2 cups of all-purpose or white whole wheat flour

Directions

1. Preheat your oven to 176.7° C (350° F).

2. Put your ginger, nutmeg, cinnamon, salt, baking soda and flour in a big bowl and mix them together.

3. Mix the brown sugar and coconut oil in a stand mixer for one or two minutes.

4. Beat the eggs one at a time into the mixture then mix the vanilla as well. The mixture may be a bit lumpy at this stage but don't worry.

5. Next, add the Greek yogurt and the apple sauce and mix well.

6. Add the dry ingredients in two installments and use the stand mixer to mix them well.

7. Use a rubber spatula to fold in the walnuts, oats and carrots and pour into the muffin tins.

8. Bake the muffins for 20 minutes.

9. Let the muffins to cool completely on a cooling rack. Drive a butter knife around the edges to remove the muffins.

10. Serve

Cabbage Hash Browns

Serves 2

Ingredients

1 tablespoon of vegetable oil

¼ small, yellow, thinly sliced onion

2 cups of shredded cabbage

Freshly ground black pepper

½ teaspoon of kosher salt

½ teaspoon of garlic powder

2 large eggs

Directions

1. Whisk together eggs, salt and garlic powder in a large bowl. Season the mixture with black pepper.

2. Add onion and cabbage to the mixture and mix them well.

3. Heat oil in a large skillet over medium heat.

4. Divide the egg and cabbage mixture into 4 patties in the pan.

5. Press with a spatula to flatten and continue cooking until tender and golden, for approximately 3 minutes each side.

Keto Cereal

Serves 3

Ingredients

¼ cup of melted coconut oil

1 large egg white

½ teaspoon of kosher salt

1 teaspoon of pure vanilla extract

1½ teaspoons of ground cinnamon

½ teaspoon of finely ground clove

2 tablespoons of chia seeds

2 tablespoons of flax seeds

¼ cup of sesame seeds

1 cup of unsweetened coconut flakes

1 cup of chopped walnuts

1 cup of chopped almonds

Cooking spray

Directions

1. Preheat your oven to 176.7° C (350° F). Then grease a baking sheet with cooking spray.

2. Mix chia seeds, flax seeds, sesame seeds, coconut flakes, walnuts, almonds together in a large bowl. Stir in the slat, vanilla, cinnamon and cloves

3. Beat the egg until it appears foamy then stir in the granola. Then add the coconut oil until the mixture is well coated

4. Pour it onto the baking sheet. Spread the mixture into an even layer.

5. Put it in the oven and bake for around 20 or 25 minutes such that it appears golden.

6. Allow it to cool completely before serving

Main Meals

Pistachio Crusted Stuffed Chicken Breasts

Serves 2

Ingredients

½ cup pistachios without shells

½ teaspoon of cumin

½ teaspoon garlic powder

½ teaspoon oregano

½ teaspoon onion powder

1 teaspoon sea salt

2 tablespoons of lemon juice

2 tablespoons cashew butter

2 tablespoons extra virgin olive oil

2 or 3 kale leaves

3 ounces almond cheese

3 tablespoons of coconut oil

4 tablespoons quinoa flakes

4 skinless and boneless chicken breasts from a free range, organic bird

Directions

1. Preheat the oven to 350° F.

2. Rinse the chicken breasts and dry them well with a paper towel. Slice into the side of each at the point where it is thickest to create a stuffing pocket.

3. Slice the roasted red pepper and kale leaves into thin slices. Shred almond cheese and stir it together with peppers and kale in a small bowl. Stuff the mixture into the chicken breast pockets you created and pin it with a toothpick to seal the stuffing.

4. Mix all herbs and spices, lemon juice, cashew butter and olive oil in a large bowl to combine them well.

5. Dip the chicken breasts in this mixture one at a time in a careful manner to avoid unpinning the toothpicks. Ensure that each breast is well coated even if it means using your hands to spread the mixture to spread the coat evenly all over the breasts.

6. Grind the pistachios with a mortar and pestle (you can also use a spice grinder). Pour it onto a large bowl alongside the quinoa flakes. Dip the coated chicken breasts into the crust mixture.

7. Heat coconut oil over medium heat in a large skillet.

8. Brown the chicken on the skillet and place it in a glass baking dish.

9. Bake the chicken for 20 or 25 minutes depending on how thick the meat was.

Kale Pesto With Squoodles (Spaghetti Squash)

Serves 10

Ingredients

1/3 cup of almonds

1 teaspoon pink Himalayan salt

1 small bunch or organic kale

1 organic spaghetti squash

2 teaspoons of freshly ground black pepper

2 cloves of garlic

3 tablespoons fresh dill

4 tablespoons of olive oil

Directions

1. Preheat the oven to 375° F (190.5° C).

2. Cut the spaghetti squash end-to-end into halves and scoop out the pulp and seeds. Place one half on a baking sheet with the cut side down. You may also bake the other side now since cooked squash stores well in the refrigerator. Bake the half for 45 minutes.

3. As the squash bakes, add all the other ingredients in a high powered blender or a food processor and blend them together.

4. Once the baked squash is tender, let it cool a bit then use a fork to separate the rinds from the fleshy strands.

5. Stir the strands with the pesto together in a large bowl.

Avocado, Quinoa And Garbanzo Bean Salad

Serves 4 to 6

Ingredients

Pepper and salt

2 tablespoons extra virgin oil

Juice from 1 lemon

1 cup of halved cherry tomatoes

1 chopped cucumber

1 large sliced avocado

1 can (15 ounces) of garbanzo beans

2 cups of cooked quinoa

Directions

1. Toss the ingredients above in a large bowl. Mix them well and serve

Avocado Chickpea Tuna Salad

Serves 4

Ingredients for the dressing

2 tablespoons freshly squeezed lemon juice

1 teaspoon minced garlic

1 tablespoon freshly chopped parsley (plus extra for serving)

¼ teaspoon salt

¼ cup olive oil

Ingredients for the salad

15 ounces canned tuna (canned in olive oil or brine)

14 ounces can of chickpeas, drained

2 large wedge-cut tomatoes

2 large peeled and pitted avocadoes

1 large cucumber, halved lengthways and sliced

½ thinly sliced red onion

Directions

1. Put all the dressing ingredients in a jar or jug and whisk them together

2. Mix the salad ingredients together in a large bowl. Toss the dressing on top

3. Season with pepper and salt

Ground Turkey Endive Roll-Ups

Serves 4

Ingredients

¼ teaspoon paprika

¼ teaspoon dried oregano

¼ teaspoon red pepper flakes

¼ teaspoon onion powder

1 teaspoon black pepper

1 teaspoon sea salt

1 teaspoon ground cumin

1 teaspoon garlic powder

1 teaspoon chilli powder

1 pound ground turkey

2 large endives

2 tablespoons coconut oil

Directions

1. Melt the coconut oil over medium heat in a large skillet.
2. Add all the spices and the ground turkey to the skillet and cook until golden brown.

3. Separate the endive leaves and spoon a few tablespoons of ground turkey into each leaf.

4. Enjoy with dairy free salsa or guacamole

Pistachio Crusted Peruvian Sea Bass And Maca

Serves 4

Ingredients

½ teaspoon black pepper

½ cup maca powder

½ cup freshly ground pistachios

1½ teaspoons of sea salt

Zest of 2 sweet limes

2 cloves of garlic

2 tablespoons of coconut oil

2 tablespoons of ghee

4 Peruvian sea bass fillets

Directions

1. Preheat the oven to 375° F.
2. Combine the garlic, coconut oil and ghee in a food processor until smooth.
3. Rub the mixture on each fillet to form an even and thick coating.

4. Heat the skillet over high heat. Let the fish fry for 2 or 3 minutes on either side then remove the fish from the heat.

5. Mix the pepper, salt, lime zest, maca powder and pistachios in a large bowl.

6. Dip each fillet in this mixture. Use both hands to ensure that the fillet is covered all around with the crumbs.

7. Put the fillets in a shallow baking dish and bake for 8 or 10 minutes until slightly flake and opaque.

8. Serve and enjoy

Ceviche

Serves 4 to 6

Ingredients

½ teaspoon organic hot sauce

½ fresh and shredded coconut meat

½ cup of finely chopped red onion

1 teaspoon freshly ground black pepper

1 teaspoon sea salt

1 pound of fresh and raw deveined, peeled shrimp without tails

2 avocados

2 medium cucumbers

2 or 3 freshly squeezed lime juice

3 Roma diced tomatoes

Directions

1. Dice the shrimp into small bitable pieces and put them in a large bowl together with the chopped onion.

2. Pour lime juice to just cover all the shrimp. Stir gently to ensure that all shrimp is doused in the juice.

3. Cover the bowl and let the shrimp marinate in the lime juice for about 20 minutes. You'll know it's ready when the flesh of the shrimp turns pink. Inspect all pieces to ensure that not one retains the initial grey color.

4. As the shrimp marinates, peel your cucumbers and cut them in halves. Scoop out the seeds with a spoon. Now chop the avocados and cucumbers together into smaller pieces.

5. Put them to a bowl and add tomatoes and coconut. Add salt, hot sauce and pepper as desired.

6. Best served alongside gluten free tortilla chips.

Crispy Sweet Potato Wedges

Serves 1 to 2

Ingredients

½ teaspoon chili flakes

½ teaspoon dried rosemary

1½ tablespoons of cold pressed, organic coconut oil

1 large organic orange-fleshed sweet potato

Pepper to taste

1 clove of minced garlic

Pink Himalayan salt

Directions

1. Preheat the oven to 425° F (218.3°)
2. Wash the sweet potato but don't peel it yet.
3. Cut it into thin wedge like pieces (for the crispiness later on). Ensure the wedges have an edge with skin about ½ inches wide.
4. Place the wedge in a large bowl and add coconut oil, pepper, garlic, salt and rosemary. Toss the bowl multiple times to ensure all the wedges are coated with spices and oil.

5. On a baking sheet, place the wedges in a single layer evenly. Bake for 15 minutes then flip the wedges over and bake again for around 8 to 10 minutes.

6. Remove them from the oven and let them cool for about 5 minutes.

7. Serve and enjoy with homemade aioli, mustard or unsweetened organic ketchup.

Honey Garlic Glazed Salmon

Serves 4

Ingredients

4 salmon fillets (patted dry with paper towels)

3 minced cloves of garlic

3 tablespoon extra virgin oil

2 tablespoons lemon juice

Freshly chopped parsley

Freshly ground black pepper

Kosher salt

1 round-sliced lemon pieces

1 teaspoon red pepper flakes

¼ cup of soy sauce

1/3 cup of honey

Directions

1. Whisk together lemon juice, soy sauce, honey and red pepper flakes in a medium bowl.

2. On a medium-high heat 2 tablespoons of oil in a large skillet.

3. Add the salmon fillet with the skin side up and season with salt and pepper.

4. Cook for about 6 minutes until it turns deep golden then flip over and add a tablespoon of oil.

5. Add garlic and cook for a minute until fragrant. Throw in the sliced lemons and honey mixture and cook until the sauce reduces by about a third. Baste sauce on the salmon.

6. Garnish with parsley and sliced lemon then serve.

Hormone Reset Crab Cakes

Serves 4 to 6

Ingredients

½ teaspoon black pepper

½ teaspoon garlic powder

½ teaspoon paprika

½ teaspoon rosemary salt

½ pound of fresh and fully cooked crab meat (use canned wild pink salmon as an alternative if crab is not in season)

1 clove of fresh garlic

1 small shallot

2 eggs

3 to 4 tablespoons of coconut oil or ghee

4 radishes

Directions

1. Pulse the garlic, shallot and radishes in the food processor until minced finely.
2. Beat the eggs in a large bowl and then add in the mixture you made above to the eggs.

3. Add all the spices and the crabmeat in the bowl and stir.

4. Heat the coconut oil (or ghee) over medium heat in a large frying pan.

5. Form small flat cakes from the crab mixture then fry each cake for about 5 to 7 minutes on either side until they appear well browned.

6. Serve over a bed of fresh greens.

Cauliflower Fried Rice

Serves 4

Ingredients

4 sliced scallions with green and white parts separated

2 large eggs

2 garlic cloves

2 tablespoons coconut aminos or tamari

2 tablespoons sesame oil

1 large or 2-3 small carrots, sliced into small bits

1 medium head of cauliflower

½ cup of frozen peas, thawed

½ small diced onion

½ teaspoon of minced ginger

Directions

1. Start by slicing the cauliflower head into two equal halves, then slice off the florets from the stem. Place the florets through the grater of a food processor and process until all cauliflower has been 'riced'.

2. Heat sesame oil on medium heat in a skillet or large wok.

3. Add ginger and garlic and sauté for 20 seconds.

4. Stir in the carrots, onions and white parts of the scallions and let it cook for 3 minutes.

5. Add peas and cauliflower rice and stir for another 2 or 3 minutes.

6. Create a well in the middle of the rice and break the eggs inside the well.

7. Stir with a spatula to scramble the eggs.

8. Once the eggs are cooked, stir everything together.

9. Finally add the green parts of the scallion and tamari then stir to combine.

10. Serve while hot

Chicken Parm Stuffed Peppers

Serves 4

Ingredients

12 ounces frozen or fresh breaded chicken, cooked and diced according to packaging instructions

4 halved bell peppers with seeds removed

3 minced cloves of garlic

3 cups shredded and divided mozzarella

1 tablespoon freshly chopped parsley (plus more for garnishing)

1½ cup marinara

½ cup swanson chicken broth

Freshly ground black pepper

Kosher salt

Pinch of crushed red pepper flakes

½ cup of freshly grated Parmesan (plus more for serving)

Directions

1. Heat your oven to 400°F

2. In a large bowl, add red pepper flakes, parsley, marinara, garlic, parmesan and 2 cups of mozzarella. Season them with salt and pepper and stir well then gently fold in chicken.

3. Spoon the mixture into the halved bell peppers and sprinkle with the remaining cup of mozzarella.

4. Add chicken broth into a baking dish and cover with foil to help the peppers to steam.

5. Put in the oven and bake for about 55 minutes or an hour until the peppers become tender.

6. Remove from oven and uncover foil then broil for 2 minutes.

7. Garnish with parmesan and parsley then serve.

Desserts

Almond Butter Fudge Bars

Serves 8

Ingredients

1 ounce of 80% sugar free chocolate or dark chocolate chips

1/8 teaspoon of xanthan gum

½ teaspoon vanilla extract

½ cup almond butter

¼ cup of heavy cream

½ teaspoon ground cinnamon

6 tablespoon of powdered erythritol sweetener

½ cup of unsalted butter (melted)

1 cup of almond flour

Directions

1. Preheat the oven to 204°C (400°F). Then line a parchment paper on a baking dish (9 by 10 inch)
2. Whisk the cinnamon, 2 tablespoons of erythritol, ¼ cup of melted butter and almond flour together until they mix well

3. Apply the mixture on the baking dish and let it bake for 10 minutes to turn golden brown

4. Whisk the remaining butter together with the almond butter, erythritol and heavy cream in a mixing bowl

5. Put in the xanthan gum and vanilla then blend them together

6. Pour a layer of fudge mixture over the now cool almond flour base. Sprinkle the top with roughly chopped sugar free or dark chocolate chips

7. Put it in the refrigerator and let it stay overnight then slice the fudge into 8 bars in the morning to serve

Chia Seed Dessert

Serves 4

Ingredients

1 tablespoon vanilla extract

1 or 2 tablespoons maple syrup to taste

½ cup chia seeds

1½ cups of dairy free milk e.g. extra creamy coconut milk

Directions

1. Add vanilla, maple syrup, chia seeds and the dairy free milk (coconut milk) to a mixing bowl. Whisk them together.

2. Cover the mixture and refrigerate it for no less than 6 hours after which the pudding will be creamy and thick. If not, add a little more chia seeds and stir then refrigerate for about n hour

3. You may eat it as it is, or you may top with a fresh fruit.

Hormone Reset Brownies

Serves 12

Ingredients for icing

¼ cup of organic hardwood derived xylitol

2 dark chocolate bars (85% or more pure cacao)

Ingredients for brownies

½ cup avocado oil

½ cup coconut sugar

½ cup organic hardwood derived xylitol

1 cup unsweetened pure cacao powder

1 tablespoon baking powder

1 or 2 tablespoons sorghum flour

2 large eggs

2 medium sweet potatoes

Directions

1. Preheat the oven to 350° F (176° C).
2. Boil 6 cups of water in a large pot.

3. Peel sweet potatoes and cut into large pieces. Put them into the boiling water and let them cook for about half an hour until they are tender.

4. Strain them and mash them in a large bowl.

5. Add cacao powder, baking powder, sorghum flour, avocado oil, coconut sugar, xylitol and eggs then stir well

6. Pour the paste into a greased 8 by 8 inch baking dish. Let it bake for around 20 to 25 minutes.

7. As it bakes, melt the chocolate in a double boiler or microwave. Add the xylitol and stir.

8. Remove the brownies from the oven and pour the mixture to form an even layer.

9. Let the melted chocolate layer cool and solidify then serve.

Hormone Reset Dips

Creamy Dairy Free Brie

Serves 6

Ingredients

2 tablespoons of raw apple cider vinegar

1 teaspoon sea salt

1 tablespoon of grass fed gelatin

1 tablespoon of soy based miso (or chick pea miso)

1 tablespoon nutritional yeast flaks

¼ cup tapioca starch and a little more for dusting

1 1/3 cup of almond milk

½ cup of melted coconut oil

Directions

1. Line ceran wrap on your mold/container or springform pan

2. Put in all the ingredients except for the apple cider vinegar in a pot and place it on medium heat. Whisk the contents for 5 minutes over the heat until you get a thick texture

3. Add the apple cider vinegar and whisk the mixture.

4. Pour the mixture into your mold or springform pan

5. Refrigerate it for 24 hours.

6. Remove the vinegar from the mold and dust it with a thick layer of tapioca flour to form your crust. When you place in the refrigerator for a few days, the crust will keep getting harder but the insides will still be soft. This is why you need to keep it chilled.

Spicy Mung-Bean Hummus

Serves 2

Ingredients

1/3 cup of water

½ teaspoon of fine grain sea salt

1 peeled and smashed clove of garlic

½ cup of tahini paste

2 tablespoons of lemon juice

1½ of cooked mung beans

Directions

1. Put all the mung beans in a food processor and pulse for a minute or so to achieve a fluffy and fine crumb.
2. Add sea salt, garlic, tahini and lemon juice then blend again for another minute. If the beans form dough looking like ball inside the processor, stop blending. Add a little splash of water at a time as you blend.
3. Keep blending until the hummus is creamy, aerated, light and smooth. Add more lemon juice or salt to your liking, if required.

Cashew Cream Cheese

Serves 8

Ingredients

½ teaspoon of salt

1 or 2 tablespoons of lemon juice

1 cup of raw cashews (soaked 4 to 8 hours in water), drained and rinsed

Stir-ins of choice e.g. veggies, roasted garlic or chives

Directions

1. Empty all ingredients (except stir-ins) into a high powered blender and blend them until smooth.
2. Add very little water to thin the paste if necessary.
3. Add the stir-ins to the processor and pulse them until they are finely chopped.
4. Accompany the cream cheese with sliced cucumbers or celery sticks.
5. If you aren't serving immediately, store in a sealed container and freeze for up to 2 months or refrigerate for 4 days.

Conclusion

We have come to the end of the book. Thank you for reading and congratulations for reading until the end.

By following the Hormone Reset Diet, you will effectively shed unwanted body fat, restore your hormones and health, rediscover the body you always dream about and feel fit and sexy.

If you found the book valuable, can you recommend it to others? One way to do that is to post a review on Amazon.

Please leave a review for this book on Amazon!

Thank you and good luck!

References

- http://www.thoughtco.com/hormones-373559
- https://www.verywellhealth.com/weight-gain-follows-hypothyroidism-treatment-3231711
- http://www.stylecraze.com/articles/hormones-responsible-for-weight-gain-in-women/?amp=1
- https://www.healthline.com/nutrition/14-ways-to-lower-insuln#section13
- http://www.foxnews.com/health/reset-your-hormones-to-lose-stubborn-pounds
- http://www.gaiam.com/blogs/discover/too-much-insulin-how-to-reset-your-metabolism
- http://www.marksdailyapple.com/leptin
- http://www.caloriecontrol.org/fructose
- http://www.foxnews.com/health/reset-your-hormones-to-lose-stubborn-pounds
- https://draxe.com/cortisol-levels/
- http://www.foxnews.com/health/reset-your-hormones-to-lose-stubborn-pounds
- https://support.storytel.se/hc/sv/article-attachments/115001883710/The-Hormon_reset_diet.pdf

- http://www.foxnews.com/health/reset-your-hormones-to-lose-stubborn-pounds

- https://www.floliving.com/the-4-ways-dairy-is-hurting-your-hormones/

- https://support.storytel.se/hc/sv/article-attachments/115001883710/The-Hormon_reset_diet.pdf

- http://www.foxnews.com/health/reset-your-hormones-to-lose-stubborn-pounds

- https://stylenik.com/the-21-day-hormone-reset-diet-was-easier-than-i-thought/

- https://support.storytel.se/hc/sv/article-attachments/115001883710/The-Hormon_reset_diet.pdf

Printed in Poland
by Amazon Fulfillment
Poland Sp. z o.o., Wrocław